Household Accidents

A Guide through Symptoms, Actions & Preventions

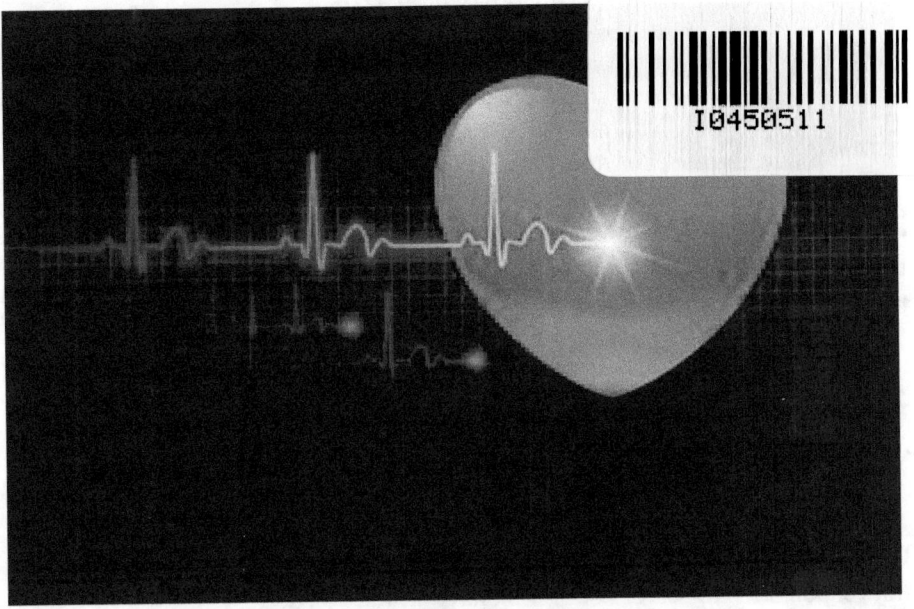

Prepping and Survival Series

M. Usman

Mendon Cottage Books

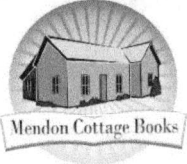

JD-Biz Publishing

Our books are available at

1. Amazon.com
2. Barnes and Noble
3. Itunes
4. Kobo
5. Smashwords
6. Google Play Books

Table of Contents

Preface

Our lives are filled with commonplace incidents and accidents as we revolve around the constant day to day activities, which have become a part of our routine. Sometimes this journey treads on some dangerous roads as we come across the domestic battles with electricity, fire, and toxic substances. Household accidents take numerous forms and sizes, but we have to tackle them and depending upon the size of the attacks we can find the defendants in our homes. We just have to know where to look and this is exactly what this book aims to do. We plan on giving you the weapons for combating these tricky and intimidating opponents.

This book deals with four basic broad categories of accidents: falling, burning, electric shocks, and accidently getting poisoned by any of the various toxic substances ever present in a common house. We cannot ensure your safety, but after going through this we are sure that depending upon the level of steps that you can endorse, you may be able to help yourself and the loved ones around you. The layout of this book is in such a manner that it introduces you with an incident and gives you its symptoms whenever you come across it and then tells you what plan of action you ought to take. Our advice does not end with your talking control of the incident, but moves on to at an even more important step which is the way to keep that incident at bay for the rest of your life. We provide you with tips and plans to prevent that accident from taking place again to protect the rest of your fate and actions.

Even though accidents are a matter of fate it is important that we try and do the best we can for our family and ourselves before leaving it to our unforeseeable future.

Chapter # 1- Introduction

Every second our future unfolds itself onto us bringing good or bad incidents in our lives. Speculation of events is mostly out of our hands, but we can try and minimize the damages that we sometimes inflict upon ourselves (unknowingly of course!). These damages that we incur in our daily routine can leave us with scarred memories, and in some serious situations, can be a source of remorse for the rest of our lives. We all have one life, lucky are the Mario brothers who can get hit by the fire, bitten by plants, and fall in ditches and come back again in a new game.

Every day people suffer accidents in their homes, accidents that sound trivial but the nature of impacts are tragic. Even though we hear these daily in our routine, incidents like falling from stairs, tripping in the bathroom, getting burned, or receiving an electric shock happen daily. These events don't put us essentially on guard because of the lax attitude people tend to show regarding them. People tend to believe that it was the mistake of others rather than the lack of precautionary steps being taken by the general public.

What this book will attempt to do is bring your attention towards these trivialities and teach you what steps you can immediately take upon in case you receive an injury in various forms. Most importantly, it will try and incorporate its motto on taking the preventive measure so that you can rather be safe than sorry. We will give various advices on each category to help in eliminating the risk from that particular incident.

Let's initiate our troubles with the most important incident that we face (have you guessed it yet?), well it's falling!

Chapter # 2- Falling

It's a weird sensation isn't it; that funny feeling in the gut and the intense helplessness when we desperately try to cling upon anything for support. Every one of us has experienced a fall, some more serious and some more comic than damaging (yes my chair got pulled away by my friend before I sat too!).

In a more serious version of things this matter has to be viewed in great detail and every step that can be taken for its prevention has to be taken leaving no stone unturned.

According to the Home Safety Council, falling is the leading cause of deaths in the home, claiming nearly 6,000 lives annually. Falls also account for 44% of all childhood injuries. Approximately 10 children in the UK die each year as a result of falling from stairs and balconies. For babies, one of the biggest threats is rolling off the side of a table, bed, or sofa and their young and eager exploration habits can lead them to troublesome areas of the house.

Kids are specially mentioned because their sustenance powers are far less when compared to adults, but the fact remains that many adults worldwide tend to slip pretty regularly as well. Now we will try to tell you how to face these falls and the correct way to get back on your feet (you are not Rocky Balboa so don't be persistent, be careful!).

The first thing to do is to catch your breath. Yes, it hurts a lot but panicking is not the solution. Try to compose yourself as much as you can.

What you are experiencing now is mixed emotions of fear, pain and, well clearly, a little bit of embarrassment. Allow yourself ample time to calm down and analyze the situation. Firstly, check your head for injuries, it's natural to be a little shaky and disoriented, but you may have a major or minor injury of the head depending upon the surface you fell on or the height from which you fell. If you have landed on a padded or soft surface from a height not greater than you, then you can apply ice to the region and see a doctor in the coming few days. In the more serious scenarios you need to go call emergency especially in case of severe bleeding.

Next, you can have a few simple checks (they are more for your conscience, let the doctor give the final opinion.)

Bleeding Check: Check for signs of bleeding, especially heavy bleeding with a pulsing flow, apply pressure directly to the wound or just above the wound (in the case of an exposed bone), and immediately call emergency medical service.

Wiggle Check: While you're down, without moving your arms and legs, wiggle your fingers and then your toes. If you can't wiggle all your digits or you experience pain while doing so, there could be some kind of muscle, nerve, or bone injury. In this scenario, kindly do not get up. Call emergency immediately or get someone to call them for you.

Pain Check: If there is no serious head injury or bleeding then move your body and limbs slowly, checking on the way for any strong pain. If the pain is strong call emergency. Also don't try to get up on your own, call someone for help. If you're alone then grab onto something and get up slowly.

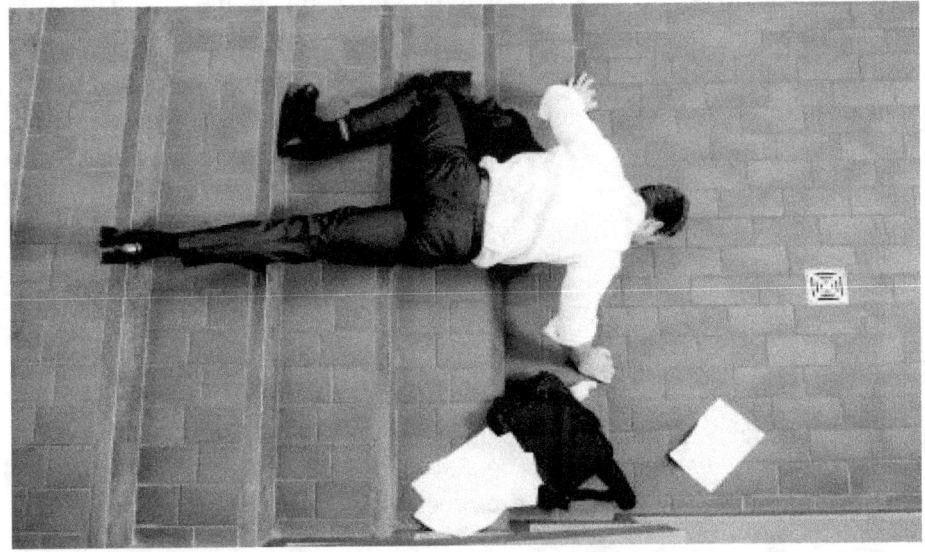

Getting back on your feet

1. Lie on your side, bend the leg gently that is on top and slowly lift yourself onto your elbows or hands.
2. Pull yourself towards a chair or any strong object, and then kneel while placing both hands firmly on the object using full support.
3. Place your stronger leg in front, holding on to the object.
4. Stand up very carefully.

All this is when the pieces are down and the tragedy has occurred, but the key stress is again on the fact that you have to look for every possible way to make sure that all this does not take in the first place.

Being safe than sorry

Very often it happens that in making sure that everything in our houses are designed to look pretty and delicate, important safety concerns are most of the time rather skimmed through or completely ignored by all of us. .

Most severe incidences occur while you are in the shower or walking on the stairs. When the deadly combination of soap and slippery tiles attack you, your poor feet do not have the ability to provide you with the safeguard. We understand that while your interior designer might recommend lavish postmodern shower arrangements, a little safety will help in the long run. Now with the level of awareness rising up, we can see that new designs are entering the markets that provide the safety value to the goods as well. For instance, additional attachments like grab bars that go with the decorum of the surroundings are now readily available in the market. Railings on the stairs are another key concern as moving on them without support is a cause for worry, because the measure of balance becomes rather unstable.

Lastly and most important, is the task of looking after the young children who solely depend upon us and have little worries regarding safety matters. Bars on windows and safety gates on stairs (the baby crawls where he wills, no boundaries!). Apart from all these precautions the essence remains to be always in the reach of the baby and to keep him/her in sight. Because disaster takes a second to incur and the consequences may last a lifetime.

So much for falling issues, yet there is a list of other important injuries that you might suffer from in your house and some of them are even more threatening. I will now turn the attention towards possibly one of the most threatening incidents that may occur, the electric current.

Chapter # 3- Electric shock

Electric sockets are the main attractions for young children, aren't they? You have to run around them each day trying to stop them from poking fingers into those curious little deadly holes unaware of the danger they carry. Next to those are something equally damaging and somehow attractive to the children, the bright red wires that they want to chew (yes all babies are hungry).

Adults also do come into contact with these devices, experimenting their way through the wires and circuits, and being the all-knowing expert, we sometimes get a little too hasty and turn out to be at the receiving end of the not so good memory of the sensation of voltage passing through our bodies. Now for the understanding of the basic essentials; there are two kinds of voltages high and low voltage. The currents in the household appliances are basically low voltage ranging from 110-220 volts while the high voltage is above 500 volts. The high voltage of 500 and above is immensely threatening while the household current is still a cause to worry, though less threatening in nature.

Secondly, other issues that matter in an electric shock are the duration, direction and the resistance of the body.

The duration of the current becomes a massive sign of worry for the victim as his survival depends on the breaking of the connection. The direction basically consists on where the flow is based. For instance, the passage from an arm to arm or an arm to leg may be more troublesome than a passage from a leg to ground, because the passage of current from an arm to arm or an arm to leg may cause damages to any vital organs like the heart.

Lastly, the resistance of the body matters a lot because tougher skin develops a greater resistance, however, damaged portions will be greatly affected, and broken areas lowers the resistances as well.

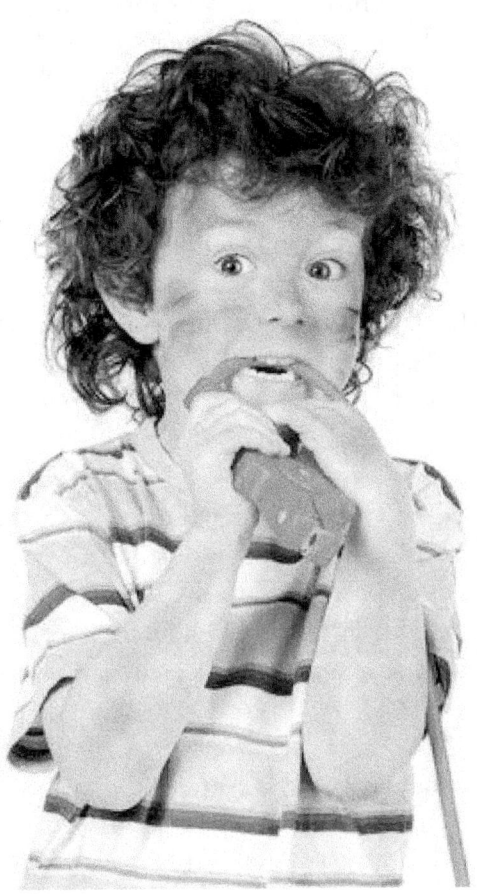

Aftermath of the shock

The trick part in the receiving of such an injury is that there might not be any physical external evidence that can bring itself to the attention of the victim; such disguised bruises are more damaging than any other form of injuries because the reaction of the attention given to the issue is delayed. Shortness of breath, chest pains, or abdominal pain can give an indication to any hidden injury.

Physical injuries may include burns. Hands, head, and heels are the most common points to check for them. Any deformity or extreme pain in limbs are indications of broken bones in the body, and may cause the contraction of muscles. In the case for children if they bite the wires, check the lips for red bruises or any burnt portion and take immediate actions.

Tackling the shocked individual

The very first thing is to break the connection of the current. DO NOT TOUCH THE PERSON RECIVING THE SHOCK, nothing can be more disastrous than this act as you will be sucked into the passage of the current as well, because all human bodies act as an electric conductor. Always seek to break the circuit or the switch by cutting off the power from the electric outlet.

After making sure that the individual is now in a stable state and the power is switched off, immediately check for a pulse and see if the individual is breathing. If the victim is found to be in a lack of state for breathing immediately apply a cardiopulmonary resuscitation (CPR). Emergency medical treatment should be instantly sought in such extreme cases because comprehensive checking is required to make sure inflicted internal damage is diagnosed.

The following circumstances require careful observation in hospitals

o   Abnormal results of ECG are found.
o   A person becomes unconscious
o   The victim is a heart patient
o   The victim is pregnant (a necessary step)

Young children who bite extension cords should be referred to an oral surgeon, or a surgeon who is experienced in the care of electric burn injuries.

Let the shock be grounded forever

The most essential step for prevention is to reduce the chance of the infants or young children to be hit by these shocks via the extension cords. Apply a cover on the unused sockets that are within the reach of young children. Their playfulness cannot and should not be stopped, but the protective measures should be increased. The use of extension cords should be limited, and the wiring should be well planned, and even more importantly, it should be regularly maintained and continuously be checked for any breakage. The broken colorful mini wires also become an attraction for the children and they are extremely dangerous.

Adolescence is an age of exploring, learning new things, and soaking yourself with experiences that teach you way much more than theory does. All these adventures should be done in a manner that is sustainable to one's health and awareness, and is an essential tool that helps us in filtering out what is better for us and what should be the limits to our experiments. This particular fine line only comes into our focus through awareness and learning. Many grownups also sometimes act foolishly by carelessly handling electrified objects near a source of water or working without turning the power off.

Chapter # 4- Poisoning

Yes, I know what you might be skeptical about this, but your house carries more poisonous objects than you might recognize or choose to believe. From overdose of medication, to substances like glue, nail polishes, or paints can carry harmful substances that might be damaging for the children. These poisons can be damaging in varying amounts for varying age groups, but all intake of such material in excess amounts, if untreated, may be really harmful to a person's health.

More than 500,000 people tend to seek emergency care in America in either deliberate or accidental poisoning and approximately 30,000 of them die each year.

How do you know the signs of poisoning?

There is huge variability in the effects of poisoning on people; some effects are instantaneous while the others may act slowly and steadily over time. Quite easily the basic factor is the age of the victim, as with age comes resistance, which varies the effects of the intake and reaction of the poison. Amounts can have a huge effect; a smaller overdose by a child can be disastrous while that same dose on an adult can be a matter of little worry.

As said, the variance in the range of symptoms is large, so let's have a look at few of the basic signs:

o   Vomiting profusely or with blood
o   Abdominal pains
o   Weakness and associated with that weakness a feeling of being
        drowsy and inactive
o   Fever chills
o   Irritation accompanied by fever
o   Experience burning sensation or pain at the affected area
o   Blurredness in the vision

o   Fits and associated seizures

o   Poisoning should not be ruled out in case of any unexplained symptom

Battling out the poison

Firstly, assess the risk of the person and see if he is unconscious or drowsy. Gently try to rouse him. If he responds that's good, but you should move him much and concentrate on what exactly is his pulse condition and make certain that his airway is open and clear. Call emergency and keep the person awake until help comes.

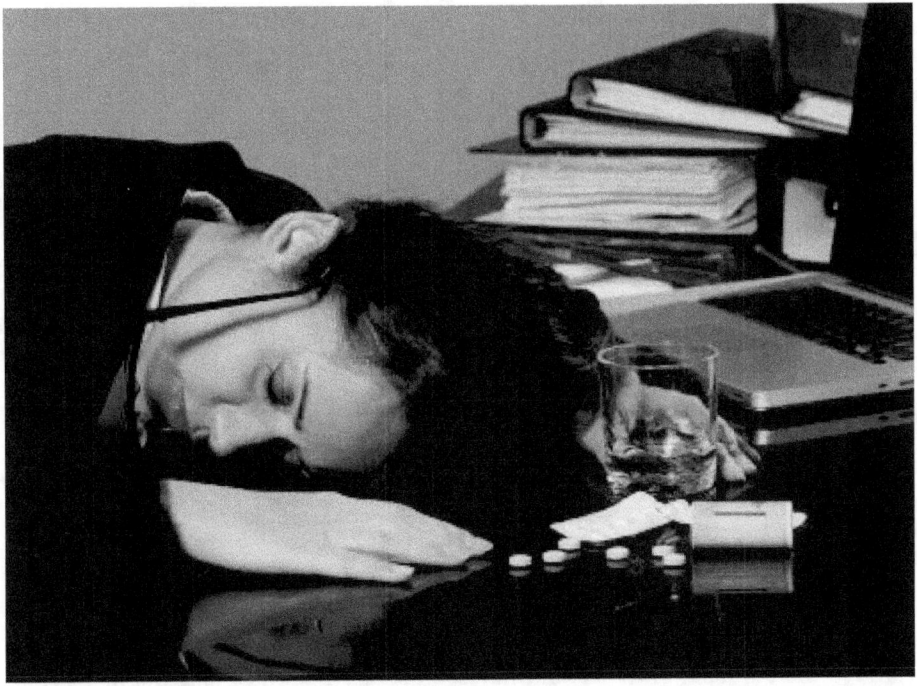

If the person does not respond, then call emergency immediately, try, and open the airway by tilting his head back and lifting his chin. If this position isn't possible, then turn him onto his back and then open the airway. If you can't feel the pulse, then start CPR.

In the scenario of poisoning, it is really helpful for the emergency staff if you can give as much information as possible, and in particular you need to know to the best of your memory the answer to the following issues:

o   What was the overdose object and even better would be if you can find the container of the item nearby.

o   The estimated time since the intake of poison.

o   If vomiting occurred or not.

o   If the incident was an accident or a deliberate attempt, this can help them in estimating the damage the person might have afflicted onto himself.

o   If you know of any illness that person has suffered or about any medication he is currently taking, inform the medical staff about them immediately. All sorts of chemicals and poisons can have different effects on the system and these can tamper with the poison.

o   If the person has pills or fluids in their mouth try to take them out, don't make him vomit as that will only cause adverse effects. The fluid or the pill residual may help the emergency staff in recognizing the poison.

If you think the person has inhaled poisonous fumes, don't expose yourself to the person's breath and use chest compressions only. You should continue at a rate of 100 to 120 compressions per minute. Continue with the compressions until the person begins breathing normally and shows signs of regaining consciousness, such as coughing, opening their eyes or until qualified help arrives.

Contamination of the skin or eyes can be caused through dust or any vapor present in the environment and they can burn or irritate you. You need to remove the clothing or any contaminated article that you think might have caused it.

The affected area should then be soaked in cold water, but you have to make sure that if the affected area is burned or infected by chemical it does not run off to other parts of the body and the seek emergency medical assistance.

Keeping the venom at bay

Keeping in mind the number of objects in our houses that have potentially harmful ingredients for our children, we have to find protective ways to keep them out of reach. We cannot get rid of them all (it would be foolish to even think about that).

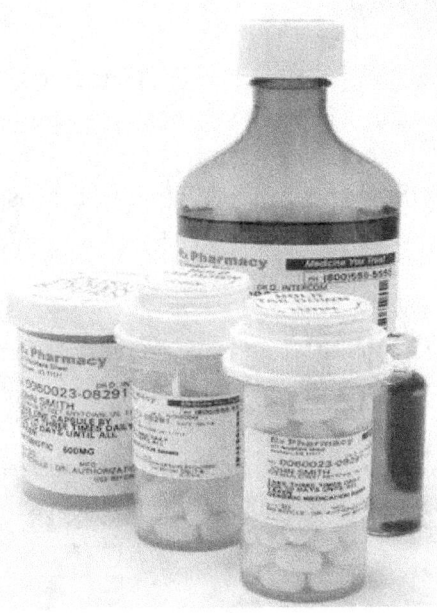

The most dangerous source of poisoning is the medications kept in our houses and the cosmetics in the dressing rooms; make sure that if you have young children in the house, that all such objects are placed in child proofed cabinets. This child proofing can be ensured via locks and bolts on the cabinets. The height of such cabinets should be raised to above that of the little children. Children are curious, naturally learn, and imitate their elders and that is the reason why you should avoid using medication in front of them, otherwise they may try to imitate your actions to adverse results. Even if you have to give your children vitamins do not explain it to them as candies or anything that is sweet, because larger amounts of these vitamins can be dangerous for them too. While purchasing medication always ask for ones with child proof capping.

Disposal of the expired medication is extremely important as throwing them away in an open disposal system can intrigue your child to take it out and eat it. Therefore it has to be ensured that their disposal container is a closed one.

Art supplies are an essential and common object found and they are mostly in use by the young children. It is an extremely essential duty at your end that you buy nontoxic art supplies.

Make sure your garage is childproofed. Store all dangerous substances like gasoline, paint, and washing fluid in locked cabinets. Know what kinds of plants you have and whether or not they are poisonous. If you do have a dangerous plant, keep it far from your child's reach or consider getting rid of it. There is never enough care that you can keep; constant vigilance is what you require.

Our next accident is one of the most common in our kitchens, burns. Burns are a common cause of injury, affecting over one million people in the United States and hospitalization of nearly 40,000 children each year. Research shows, however, that more than 80 percent of burns to children are avoidable and may be stopped by taking efficient and effective measures.

Chapter # 5- Household burns

Approximately two million American households suffer burn injuries and around seventy thousand of these cases require hospitalization.

According to Dr. David Wilcox "Burns are one of the leading causes of accidental injuries in childhood, and the greatest tragedy is that many of these could have been prevented. Fortunately, there are steps you can take to protect your family and avoid a trip to the emergency department."

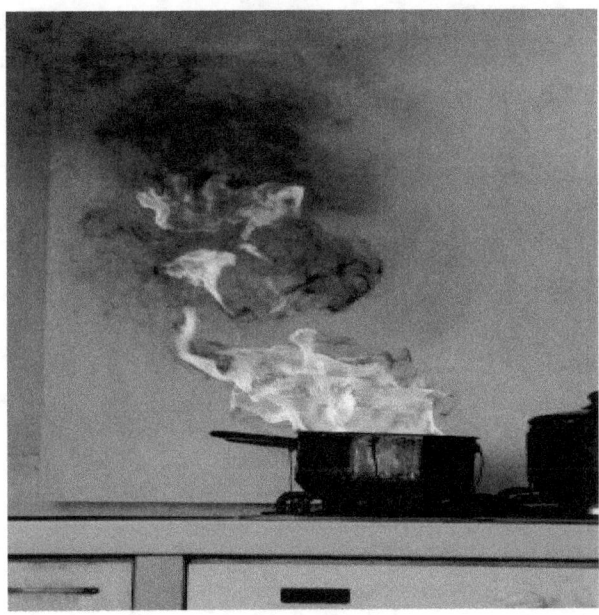

Know your burns

Burns are classified by three different degrees. In the first degree burns only the outer layer of the skin is affected and the area under influence of the burns is in pain and turns red but no blistering occurs; all minor burns are kept under this category. The second degree burns have deeper reach, the leakage of fluids caused by the burning may lead to damaged blood vessels, and blistering occurs on the affected area. If the damaged area is large or infected then these burns can be disastrous in nature. Especially seek medical assistance if the burnt areas include hands, feet, face, or genitals.

Signs of extreme danger are indicated by the third degree burns. They affect both the outer and the inner layers of the skin and damages the blood vessels, muscles and even bones. The burnt area takes the appearance of black or white and it is apparently painless as the nerves have been damaged and they do not pass the signals to brain. This is the worst case scenario for burning cases and immediate medical assistance has to be sought.

Adding relief to fire

Yes an image of a cartoon catching fire on its buttocks and running around in panic mode may be hilarious to look at, but seriously do not follow their footsteps. As with all the accidents remaining calm is the very first and important step that one has to take, because you need your brain to think and remember what you read in this book to overcome the situation.

The following symptoms are those in which seeking medical attention is an absolute necessity

o   Initiation of fever after the burns.
o   Foul smelling drainage.
o   Excessive swelling on the burnt area of your body.
o   Excessive redness of the skin.
o   Blisters filled with brown or greenish fluids.
o   If the burn does not heal in 10-12 days.

Here are several different things that can help you (apply the one that appears first on your mind)

o   Cold water is the very first thing that enters your mind, isn't it? It's rather instantaneous and impulsive of your brain to think of that and yes you can immediately apply running water over the burned area and repeat the remedy every few hours. APPLYING ICE TO THE BURNED AREA IS A BAD IDEA. Ice restricts the blood flow in the burned portion of your body and can eventually damage delicate tissues.
o   Raw potato has anti-irritating and soothing properties and that makes it a great choice to apply on burnt areas. It alleviates pain and

the chances that you'll have blisters are greatly lowered. The best method is to cut off a slice and rub it, ensuring that the juice flows over the damaged area.

o   Aloe Vera has astringent, tissue-healing, and painkilling properties. What you need to do before applying it is that you have to rinse the affected area with cold water and then rub the aloe Vera leaf .In case you do not have the leaf apply Aloe Vera gel on the burnt area.

o   Coconut Oil and Lemon Juice concoction is an excellent remedy as well. Rich in vitamin E and fatty acids coconut oil offers anti-fungal, anti-oxidizing, and anti-bacterial properties. While lemon juice helps in naturally lightening the scars.

o   Honey is an effective disinfectant and can help in healing burns by drawing fluids out of the tissues and it cleans up the burnt area. Apply honey on a gauze bandage and change it three to four times a day.

o   Black Tea Bags helps by drawing the heat out of the burn and relive pain. All you have to do is to place three teabags in cold water and let them sit for a few minutes then dab them gently on your wound.

o   Rinsing the burnt area with vinegar after diluting it with water is another excellent remedy for this issue. Instead of rinsing the burnt area, a diluted amount of vinegar can be soaked in a cloth and can be kept over the damaged region.

Keeping your distance with the blazing fames

Cooking is predominantly the action that attracts these burns as fire is the main element to food. While cooking it becomes necessary to take particular actions so that one can escape the wrath of fire. You can keep the pot handles towards the rear of the stove and every pot placed on fire has to be closely watched like troops on a battlefield. The food items and their closeness to the young members of our family have to be avoided at all costs. Not only should you check the temperature of the food or beverage that you are handing out to the young ones, we also have to take care that those items are not left by them at the edges of a table.

Lighters, matches, and electric outlets can be a devil in disguise in the wrong hands and a blessing in another. It is absolutely essential to keep them away from the reach of children and keep the safety caps and lids on. Fire extinguishers are your guardian angels in the scenario of a fire breaking out and it is advisable that you keep one on every floor of your house, especially the kitchen, because adding water to a grease fire will act literally as adding fuel to it and will spread it.

Add new technologies like smoke detectors in your house to ensure its safeguard and always remember the key thing if you catch fire, do not run, drop to the floor instantaneously and roll while covering your face and hands to smother the flames.

Chapter # 6- Conclusion

So many symptoms, plans of actions, and methods of prevention are not given here to dazzle you or bamboozle you with so many theories, but are there so that we can provide you with assistance at your moment of dire need.

Tragedies unfold in front of us in literally moments, the blink of an eye is all it takes, and we can do nothing about it (at least until they hurry up with the time machine). But we can alter the paths by taking measures we sometimes choose to ignore or do not give preference over beautification of our houses or simply because we feel that they are mere trivialities. Truth is, we need to remain prepared, and we need to know what we can do to combat these scenarios. We need to know what we are up against so that we are not at a disadvantage when the calamity strikes, but have it all under control because we are prepared and we have the understanding of how to handle these situations for our and our family's betterment. Knowledge is what comes to our rescue when we need the assistance in any troubled situation.

How to Do CPR?

- **Step # 1:** Immediately call emergency services without wasting a second.
- **Step # 2:** Your safety comes first. Check the affected person and the surroundings for any danger. Don't go near the affected person if you suspect any danger (falling bricks will injure you too and then there we'll be no one to help you both) and wait for the help to come.
- **Step # 3:** Lay down the person on a hard surface. If you're doing CPR on a mattress or foam then it's never going to work.
- **Step # 4:** Sit down on your knees so that you're on the right side of the affected person.
- **Step # 5:** Check the see if he is conscious or not. Call him to see if he responds. If not then pinch him hard on his shoulders. If he doesn't respond at all then check him for carotid pulse.
- **Step # 6:** Check the inside of the affected person's mouth for any object or poison. Clear his mouth with the help of a cloth. Try and open the airway by tilting his head back and lifting his chin. Cover the mouth with a cloth and breathe in forcefully. If his chest raises as you breathe the air in then you're doing it right. Repeat this process twice.
- **Step # 7:** Now sitting on the right side, place your right hand over your left (opposite if you're a left hander) and place both over the left side of the chest (where the heart is).
- **Step # 8:** Stay firm on your knees and push the chest down forcefully, don't hold back. Use your entire arm and back to push down the chest. Make sure that your elbows remain locked and they don't move. Repeat the process 30 times and then give another breathe by the same process as mentioned above. You've completed one cycle.
- **Step # 9:** Complete the entire cycle 5 times and after that check for the pulse.
- **Step # 10:** If the person comes back to consciousness or you feel a pulse then stop the CPR, otherwise keep repeating the cycle until help comes.

References

http://www.emedicinehealth.com/electric_shock/page2_em.htm#electric_sh
ock_causes

http://www.emedicinehealth.com/electric_shock/page4_em.htm#when_to_s
eek_medical_care

http://www.emedicinehealth.com/electric_shock/page3_em.htm#electric_sh
ock_symptoms

http://www.emedicinehealth.com/electric_shock/page8_em.htm#electric_sh
ock_prevention

http://www.merckmanuals.com/home/injuries_and_poisoning/electrical_and
_lightning_injuries/electrical_injuries.html

http://www.bupa.co.uk/individuals/health-information/directory/p/poisoning

http://www.whattoexpect.com/toddler/childhood-injuries/childhood-
poisoning.aspx

http://www.emergencycareforyou.org/EmergencyManual/WhatToDoInMedi
calEmergency/Default.aspx?id=262

http://my.clevelandclinic.org/healthy_living/safety/hic_household_chemical
s_whats_in_my_house.aspx

http://health.howstuffworks.com/wellness/natural-medicine/home-
remedies/home-remedies-for-burns.htm

http://www.top10homeremedies.com/home-remedies/home-remedies-for-
minor-burns.html/3

http://tipnut.com/minor-kitchen-burns/

http://www.emergencycareforyou.org/yourhealth/injuryprevention/default.aspx?id=25990

http://www.phac-aspc.gc.ca/seniors-aines/publications/public/injury-blessure/falls-chutes/index-eng.php

http://money.usnews.com/money/blogs/the-home-front/2009/08/31/the-top-5-causes-of-accidental-home-injury-deathsand-how-to-prevent-them

http://www.nhs.uk/Conditions/Accidents-to-children-in-the-home/Pages/How-to-prevent-accidents.aspx

http://www.parentcare101.com/Articles/WhatToDoAfterAFall.html

Author Bio

Muhammad Usman is a distinguished medical graduate of Allama Iqbal medical college (AIMC). He is a professional writer who has been in the field for more than 4 years. During this time he has produced 10,000+ articles, blogs, and eBooks on various niches related to diseases, health, fitness, nutrition, and well-being. He is a regular contributor to several journals related to medicine and surgery. He is the editor of several journals and newspapers.

Check out some of the other JD-Biz Publishing books

Gardening Series on Amazon

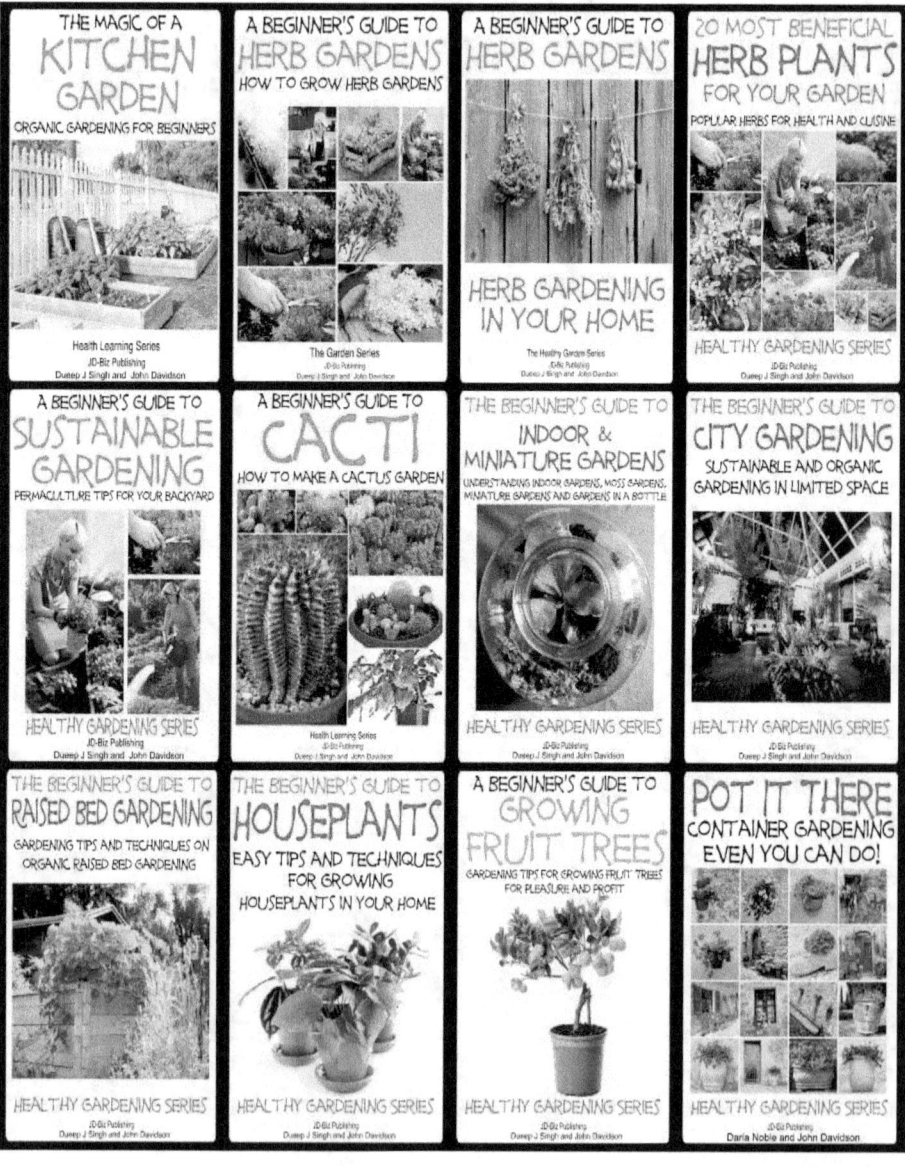

Health Learning Series

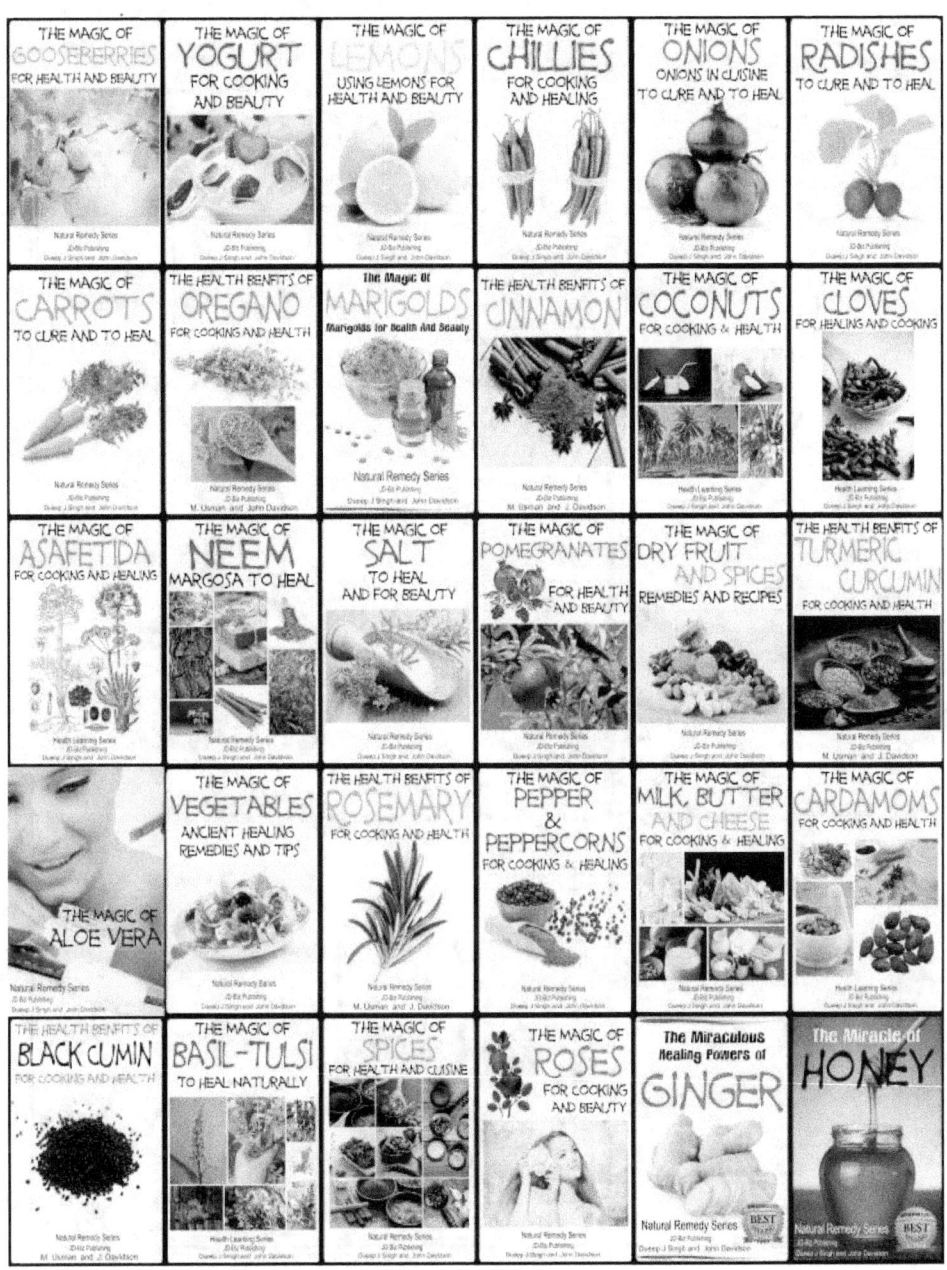

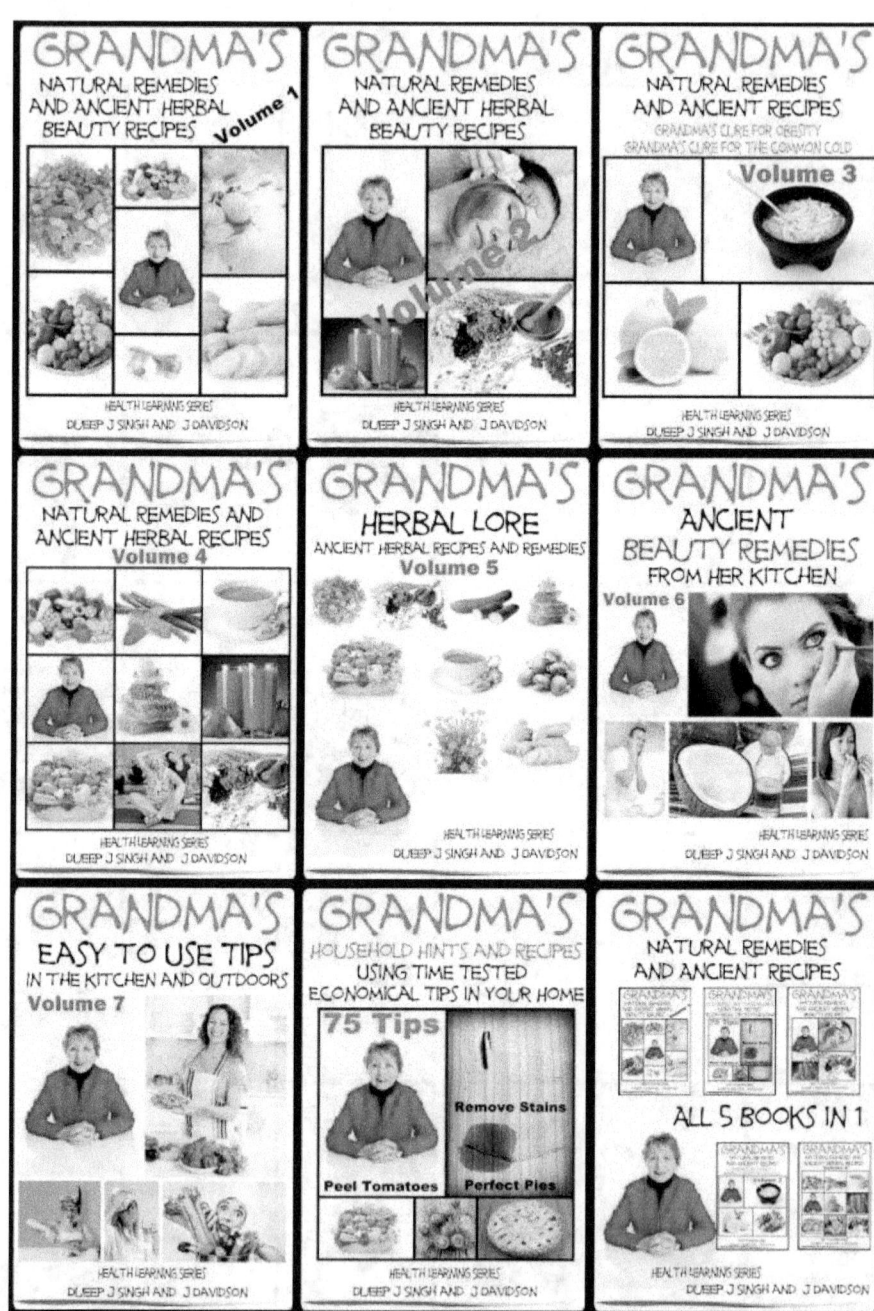

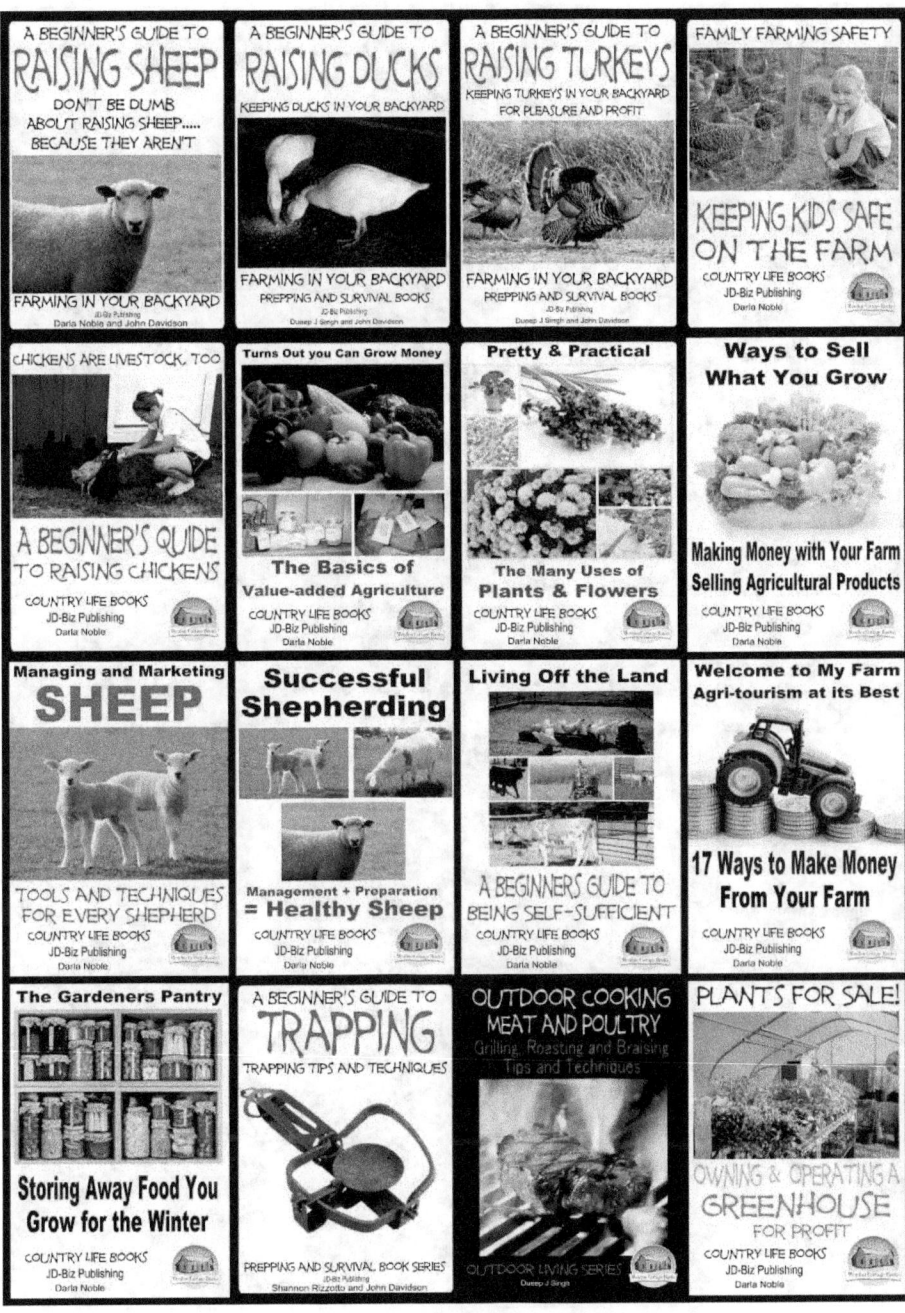

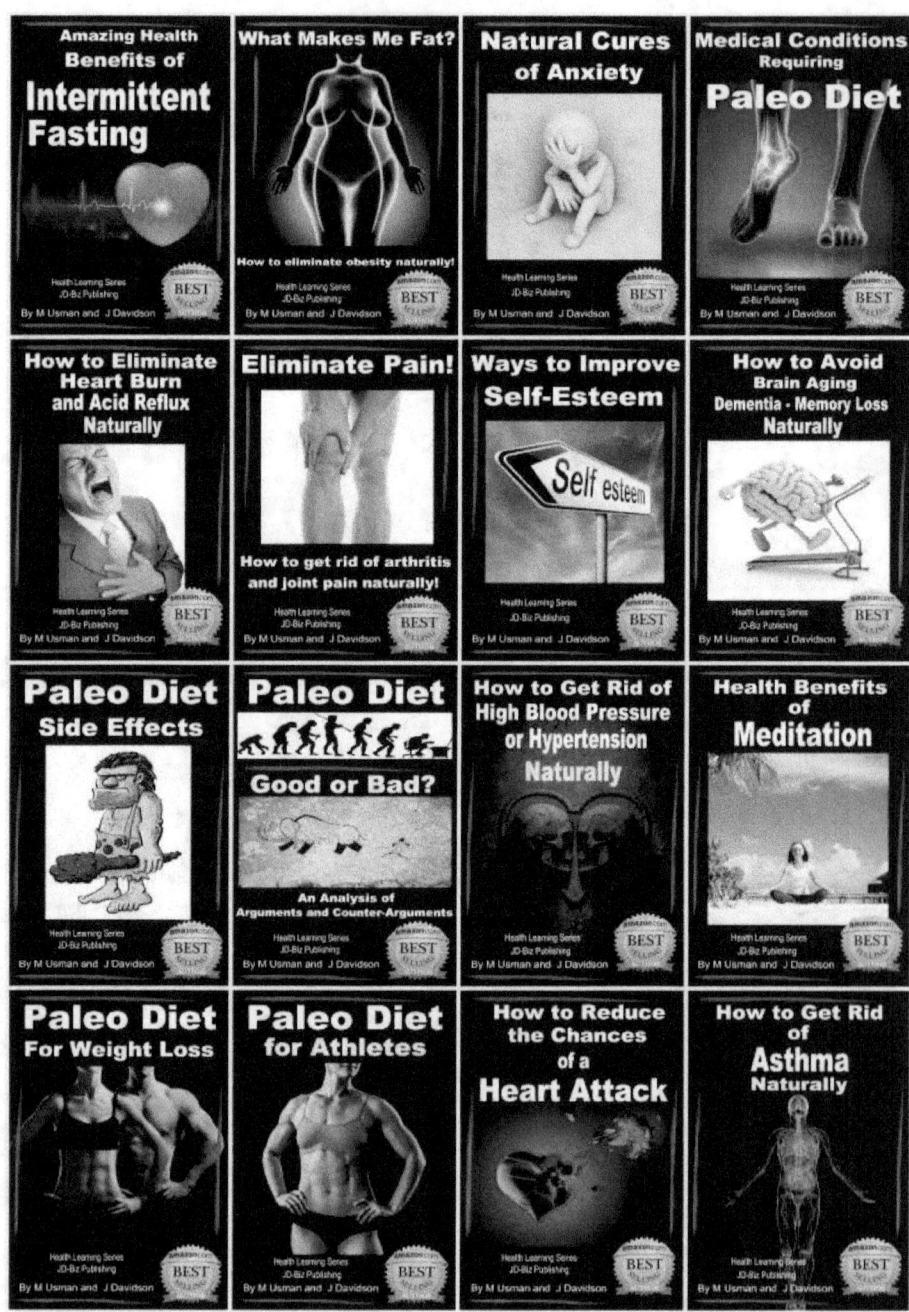

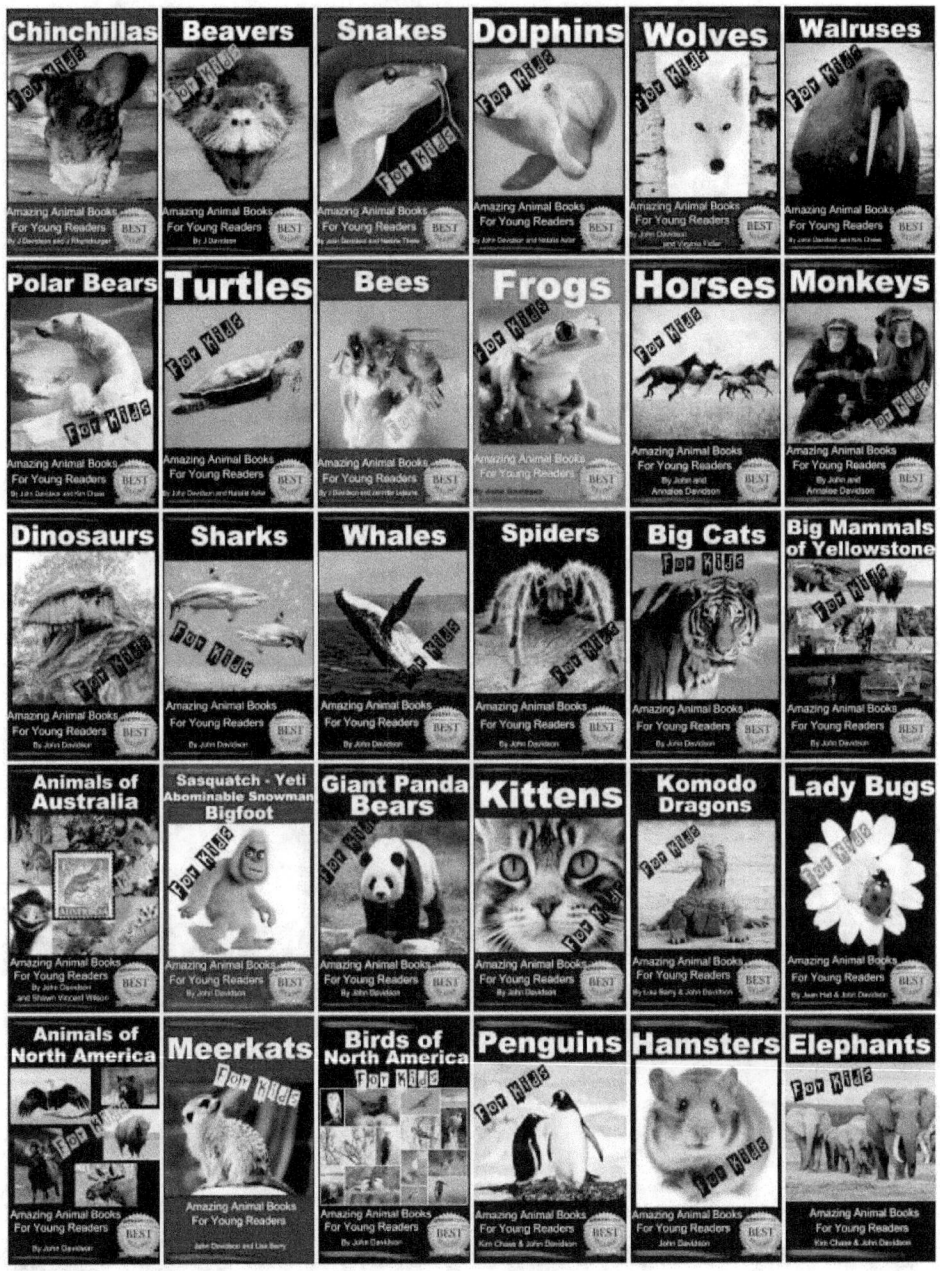

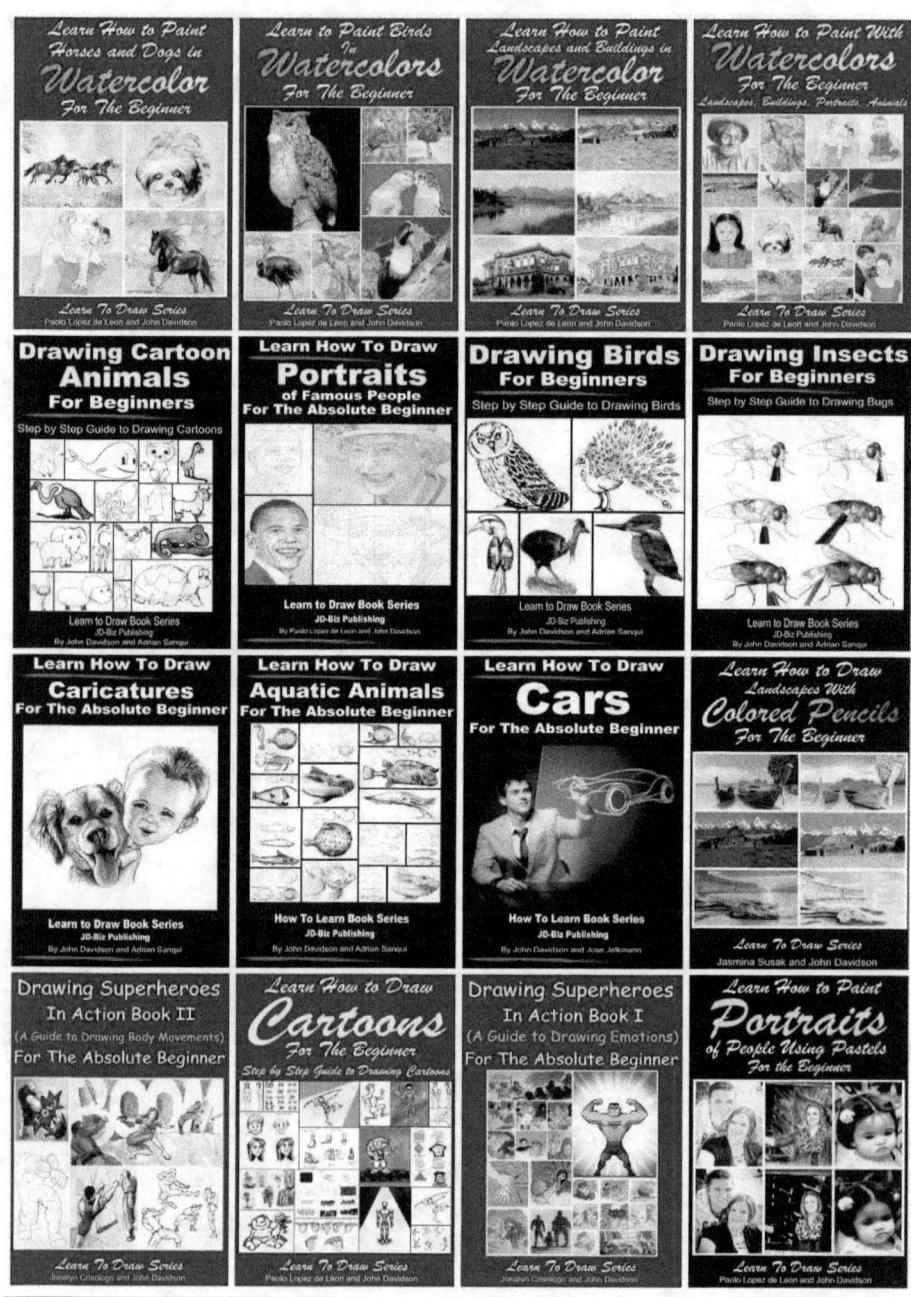

How to Build and Plan Books

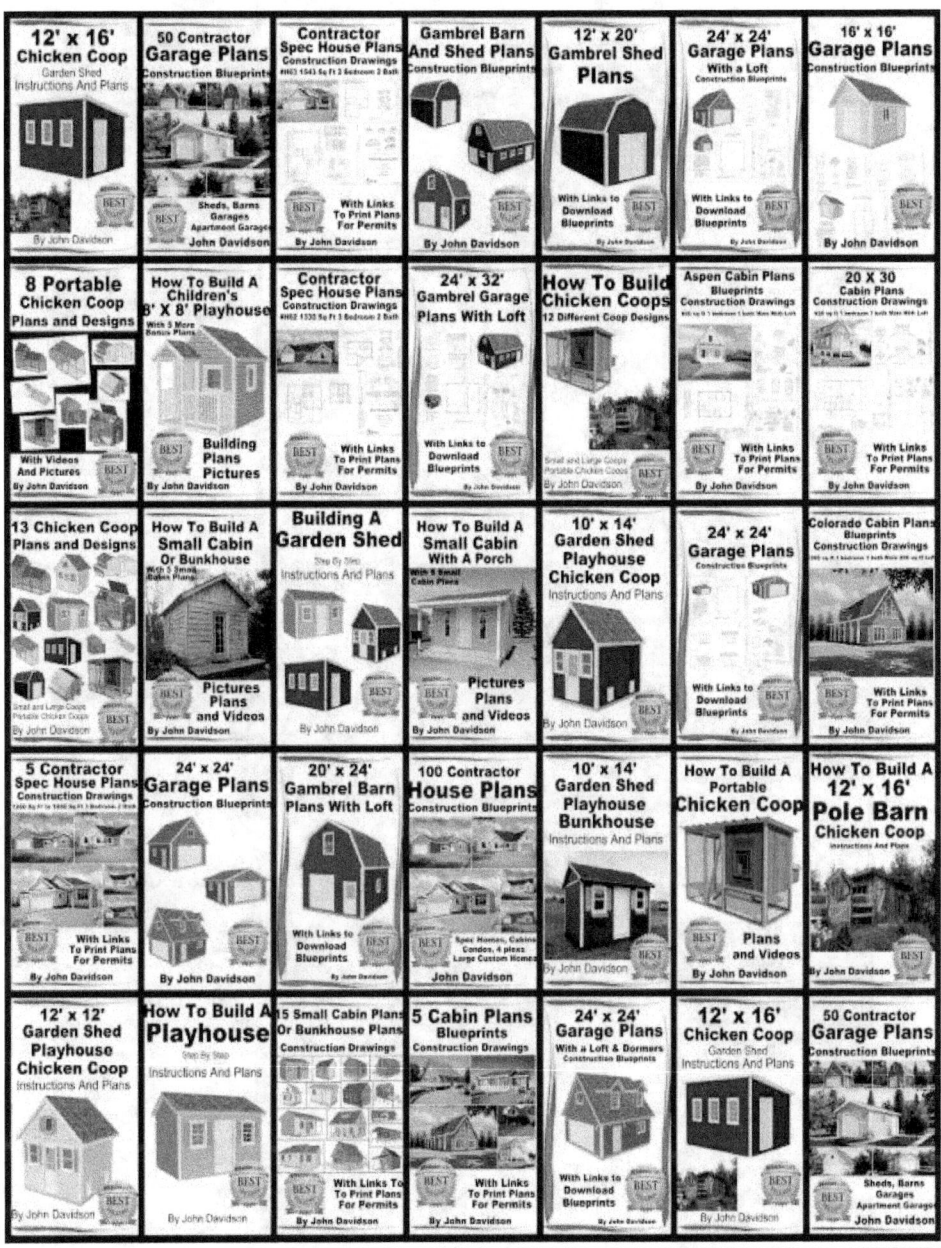

Entrepreneur Book Series

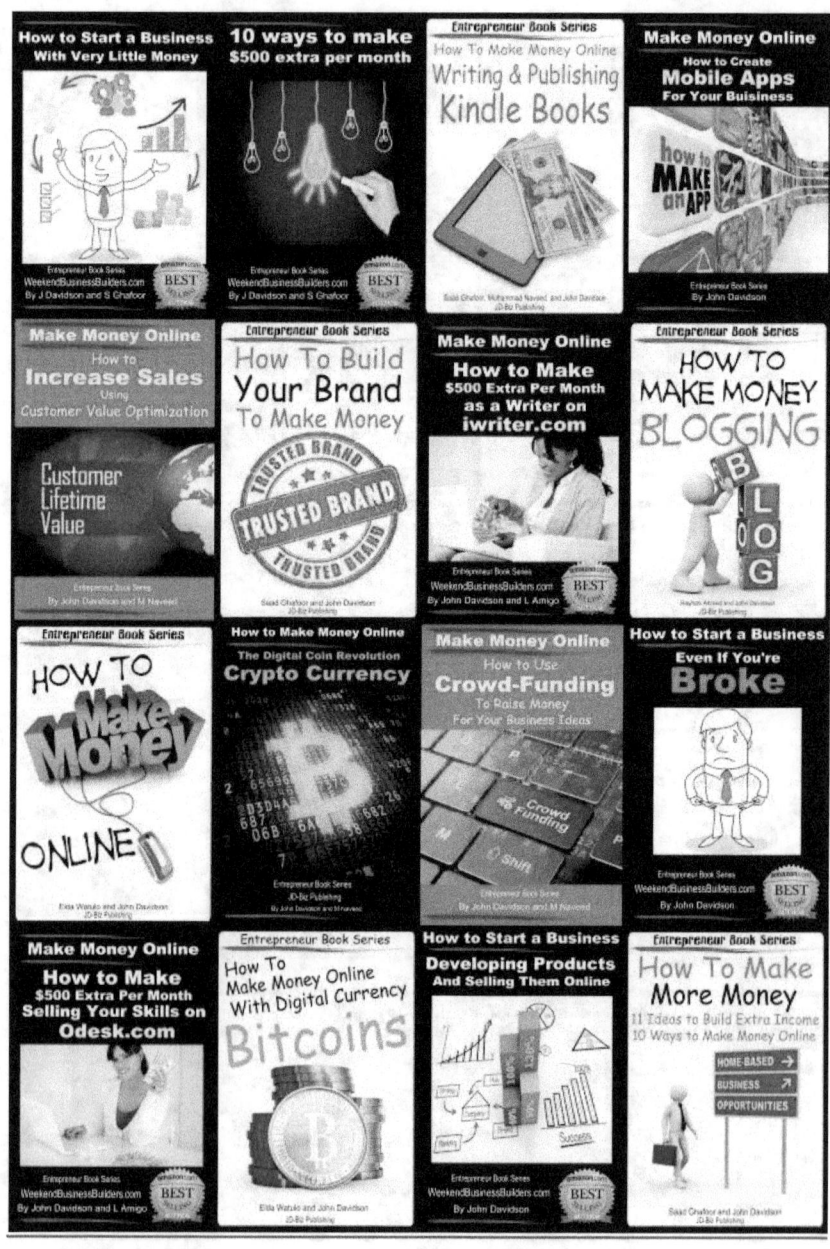

Our books are available at

1. Amazon.com

2. Barnes and Noble

3. Itunes

4. Kobo

5. Smashwords

6. Google Play Books

Publisher

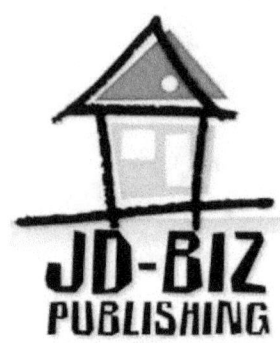

JD-Biz Corp

P O Box 374

Mendon, Utah 84325

http://www.jd-biz.com/

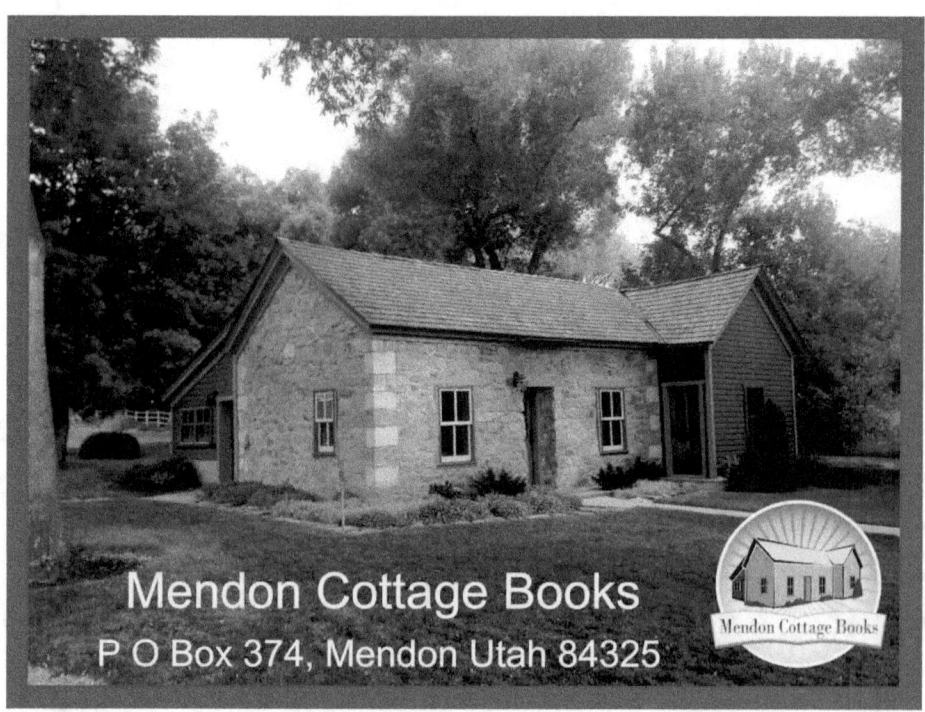

Mendon Cottage Books
P O Box 374, Mendon Utah 84325

www.ingramcontent.com/pod-product-compliance
Lightning Source LLC
Chambersburg PA
CBHW061931280526
45787CB00004B/1560